No sugar diet for beginners

Navigating the No-Sugar Diet for Beginners

Dr. Rose Shineman

No sugar diet for beginners
Navigating the No-Sugar Diet for Beginners
Dr. Rose Shineman

No sugar diet for beginners
Navigating the No-Sugar Diet for Beginners
Dr. Rose Shineman
Copyright
Introduction
No sugar diet for beginners
Natural sweeteners
Choosing Whole foods
Difference in Whole foods and processed foods
Whole Foods:
Processed Foods:
Choosing a Balanced Approach:
Gradual reduction approach
Understanding the impact of sugar on health
Health benefits of no sugar diet
Meal plan
No sugar diet drinks and beverages

Copyright

© [2024] by [Dr. Rose Shineman]

This guide is designed to provide general information on adopting a no-sugar diet for beginners and is not intended to be a substitute for professional medical advice, diagnosis, or treatment. Always seek the advice of your physician or other qualified health provider with any questions you may have regarding a medical condition. Never disregard professional medical advice or delay in seeking it because of something you have read in this guide.

Introduction

In a quaint town nestled between rolling hills and sun-kissed orchards, lived Emma, a woman with an unyielding passion for health and well-being. Emma's journey toward a no-sugar diet began not as a drastic transformation but as a gentle awakening to the power of mindful eating.

It all started one crisp morning when Emma found herself standing in the bustling aisles of her local grocery store, carefully examining the labels of the food she held in her hands. As her fingers traced the fine print, she realized the omnipresence of sugar—hidden in cereals, lurking in sauces, and even masquerading as "healthy" in seemingly innocent yogurt containers.

Curiosity turned into a quest as Emma delved into the science behind sugar and its profound impact on health. Armed with newfound knowledge, she embarked on a journey toward a no-sugar diet, not as a stringent rule but as a gentle transition to a lifestyle that prioritized nourishment over empty calories.

Emma discovered the beauty of whole foods – the vibrant colors of fresh fruits and vegetables, the earthy richness of whole grains, and the satisfying crunch of nuts and seeds. Her kitchen became a canvas where she experimented with natural sweeteners like honey and stevia, finding delightful alternatives that satisfied her sweet tooth without compromising her commitment to health.

As Emma embraced this journey, she noticed changes beyond the physical. Her energy levels soared, her skin glowed with vitality, and the fog that once clouded her mind lifted. Friends and neighbors began to notice the transformation, and Emma found herself becoming a source of inspiration for those seeking a similar path to wellness.

The story of Emma's no-sugar journey is not one of deprivation but of empowerment—a testament to the transformative power of mindful, intentional choices. It's a journey that invites everyone, beginners and seasoned health enthusiasts alike, to reconsider their relationship with sugar and embark on a path where every meal is a celebration of whole, nourishing foods.

In the heart of that charming town, Emma's story became a whisper of change, a gentle reminder that every journey toward a healthier, sugar-conscious life begins with a single, mindful step.

No sugar diet for beginners

Embarking on a no-sugar diet can have various health benefits, from improved weight management to better blood sugar control. Here are some tips for beginners:

1. Understand Hidden Sugars:
   - Learn to identify hidden sugars in processed foods by checking ingredient labels. Look for terms like sucrose, high fructose corn syrup, and other sugar aliases.
2. Choose Whole Foods:
   - Focus on whole, unprocessed foods like fruits, vegetables, lean proteins, and whole grains. These foods contain natural sugars along with essential nutrients and fiber.
3. Gradual Reduction:
   - Instead of quitting sugar abruptly, consider reducing your intake gradually. This approach can make the transition more manageable and sustainable.
4. Read Nutrition Labels:

- Pay attention to nutrition labels when shopping. Choose products with little to no added sugars. Be aware that some seemingly healthy items, like certain yogurts or sauces, can contain hidden sugars.

5. Opt for Natural Sweeteners:

   - If a sweetener is necessary, consider using natural options like stevia, monk fruit, or erythritol. These alternatives provide sweetness without the same impact on blood sugar.

6. Mindful Eating:

   - Practice mindful eating to develop a better understanding of your body's hunger and fullness cues. This can help prevent unnecessary snacking on sugary items.

7. Stay Hydrated:

   - Drink plenty of water throughout the day. Sometimes, feelings of hunger can be confused with dehydration. Staying hydrated may reduce sugar cravings.

8. Plan Balanced Meals:

   - Plan well-balanced meals that include a combination of protein, healthy fats, and complex carbohydrates. This can help stabilize blood sugar levels and reduce sugar cravings.

9. Healthy Snack Options:

    ○ Choose nutritious snacks such as fresh fruit, veggies with hummus, or a handful of nuts. These alternatives can satisfy your sweet or savory cravings without resorting to sugary treats.

10. Cook at Home:

    ○ Cooking meals at home gives you better control over the ingredients. You can experiment with herbs and spices to add flavor without relying on sugar.

11. Educate Yourself:

    ○ Learn about the impact of sugar on your health. Understanding the reasons for reducing sugar can motivate and empower you to make healthier choices.

12. Accountability and Support:

    ○ Share your no-sugar journey with friends or family members. Having a support system can make the process more enjoyable and provide accountability.

13. Treat Yourself Occasionally:

    ○ Allow yourself occasional treats or desserts to prevent feeling deprived. Moderation is key, and occasional indulgences can help you stick to the overall no-sugar plan.

Remember, making dietary changes takes time and patience. It's essential to listen to your body and find a balance that works for you. Consulting with a healthcare professional or a registered dietitian can provide personalized guidance based on your specific health needs and goals.

Natural sweeteners

Natural sweeteners can be a healthier alternative to refined sugars and artificial sweeteners. Here are some common natural sweeteners:

1. Honey:
   - A natural sweetener produced by bees, honey contains various antioxidants and has a distinctive flavor. It's important to note that honey is still a form of sugar and should be used in moderation.
2. Maple Syrup:
   - Extracted from the sap of maple trees, maple syrup provides a sweet, rich flavor. Choose pure maple syrup without added sugars or artificial ingredients.
3. Agave Nectar:

- Derived from the agave plant, agave nectar is sweeter than sugar, so smaller amounts can be used. It has a low glycemic index, making it a potential option for those managing blood sugar levels.

4. Dates:
   - Dates are a natural sweetener packed with fiber and essential nutrients. They can be blended into date paste and used in baking or as a sweetener in various dishes.

5. Stevia:
   - Extracted from the leaves of the Stevia rebaudiana plant, stevia is a zero-calorie sweetener that is much sweeter than sugar. It's available in liquid, powder, or granulated form.

6. Monk Fruit:
   - Monk fruit sweetener comes from the monk fruit and is known for its intense sweetness without calories. It can be used as a sugar substitute in various recipes.

7. Coconut Sugar:
   - Made from the sap of coconut palm trees, coconut sugar has a similar taste to brown sugar. It contains some nutrients and has a lower glycemic index compared to regular sugar.

8. Molasses:

   - Molasses is a byproduct of the sugar refining process and is rich in iron and other minerals. Blackstrap molasses, in particular, is a more concentrated form.

9. Xylitol:

   - Xylitol is a sugar alcohol found in various fruits and vegetables. It is often used as a sugar substitute and is known for its ability to prevent tooth decay.

10. Erythritol:

    - Another sugar alcohol, erythritol is naturally found in certain fruits. It is low in calories, does not affect blood sugar levels, and has a similar taste to sugar.

When using natural sweeteners, moderation is key, as they still contribute to overall sugar intake. It's also crucial to consider individual health conditions, such as diabetes, when incorporating these sweeteners into your diet. Consulting with a healthcare professional or a registered dietitian can help you make informed choices based on your specific needs and health goals.

Choosing Whole foods

Whole foods are foods that are as close to their natural state as possible, minimally processed, and free from additives or artificial substances. They are often considered nutritious choices because they retain their original nutrient content and provide essential vitamins, minerals, fiber, and other beneficial compounds. Here are some examples of whole foods:

1. Fruits and Vegetables:
   - Apples, bananas, berries, oranges, spinach, kale, broccoli, carrots, and other fresh produce.
2. Whole Grains:
   - Brown rice, quinoa, oats, barley, whole wheat, and other whole grains that haven't undergone extensive processing.
3. Legumes:
   - Beans, lentils, chickpeas, and other legumes are excellent sources of protein, fiber, and various nutrients.
4. Nuts and Seeds:
   - Almonds, walnuts, chia seeds, flaxseeds, and sunflower seeds are nutrient-dense whole foods.
5. Lean Proteins:

- o Chicken, turkey, lean beef, fish, tofu, and other minimally processed protein sources.

6. Dairy:

- o Milk, yogurt, and cheese in their natural forms, without added sugars or artificial ingredients.

7. Eggs:

- o Eggs provide a rich source of protein and various essential nutrients.

8. Herbs and Spices:

- o Fresh or dried herbs like basil, oregano, and spices such as cinnamon, turmeric, and ginger enhance flavor without adding calories or processed ingredients.

9. Healthy Fats:

- o Avocado, olives, nuts, and seeds contain healthy fats that contribute to overall well-being.

10. Fish:

- o Fatty fish like salmon, mackerel, and sardines provide omega-3 fatty acids and are considered whole, unprocessed foods.

11. Tubers:

- Sweet potatoes and regular potatoes are nutritious tubers that can be prepared in various ways.

12. Whole-Milk Products:

- In moderation, whole-milk dairy products like full-fat yogurt or cheese can be part of a balanced diet.

13. Unprocessed Meats:

- Unprocessed cuts of meat, such as chicken breasts, turkey, or lean beef, without added preservatives or flavorings.

14. Whole-Grain Products:

- Foods made from whole grains, like whole wheat bread or brown rice, that retain the fiber and nutrients present in the original grain.

Whole foods form the foundation of a healthy, balanced diet and are associated with various health benefits, including better weight management, improved digestion, and a reduced risk of chronic diseases. Incorporating a variety of whole foods into your meals supports overall well-being and provides a diverse range of nutrients.

Difference in Whole foods and processed foods

Whole foods and processed foods differ significantly in their composition, nutritional content, and impact on health. Here are key distinctions between the two:

Whole Foods:

1. Definition:

   - Whole foods are in their natural, unprocessed state, containing one ingredient or very few ingredients.

2. Nutrient Density:

   - Whole foods are nutrient-dense, providing essential vitamins, minerals, fiber, and other beneficial compounds in their natural form.

3. Minimal Processing:

   - These foods undergo minimal processing, retaining their original nutritional content. Processing is typically limited to cleaning, cutting, or cooking.

4. Examples:

   - Fruits, vegetables, whole grains, lean meats, nuts, seeds, and dairy products without added sugars or preservatives.

5. Health Benefits:

    o Whole foods are associated with various health benefits,
      including better digestion, weight management, and a reduced
      risk of chronic diseases.

6. Digestible Fiber:

    o Whole foods often contain fiber, promoting digestive health,
      regulating blood sugar levels, and contributing to a feeling of
      fullness.

Processed Foods:

1. Definition:

    o Processed foods undergo significant alterations from their
      original state, often involving the addition of preservatives,
      sweeteners, colors, and other additives.

2. Nutrient Content:

    o Processing can strip foods of some nutrients, and certain
      additives may be included for taste, texture, or shelf life.

3. Extent of Processing:

- ○ Processed foods range from minimally processed items (like frozen vegetables) to highly processed products (like sugary snacks or fast food).

4. Examples:

   - ○ Breakfast cereals, packaged snacks, sugary beverages, fast food, and convenience meals are examples of processed foods.

5. Health Considerations:

   - ○ Highly processed foods are often associated with health concerns, including excess calorie consumption, added sugars, unhealthy fats, and a potential lack of essential nutrients.

6. Convenience vs. Nutrition:

   - ○ While processed foods are convenient, they may not provide the same nutritional benefits as whole foods. They can contribute to a less diverse and nutrient-poor diet if consumed excessively.

Choosing a Balanced Approach:

- Balancing Both:

- A healthy diet often involves a balance. While whole foods form
    the foundation, some minimally processed items can be part of
    a balanced diet.
  - Reading Labels:
    - When choosing processed foods, reading labels is essential to
      identify additives, preservatives, and added sugars. Opt for
      items with shorter ingredient lists and recognizable
      components.
  - Limiting Ultra-Processed Foods:
    - Limiting the intake of ultra-processed foods, which often contain
      high levels of additives and low nutritional value, is generally
      recommended for overall health.

In summary, focusing on a diet rich in whole foods while being mindful of processed food choices can contribute to overall well-being. Prioritizing nutrient-dense, minimally processed options supports optimal health and nutrition.

Gradual reduction approach

The gradual reduction approach to a no-sugar diet is a thoughtful and sustainable strategy that allows individuals to ease into the lifestyle change without feeling overwhelmed. Here's a step-by-step guide:

1. Assessment:

- Begin by assessing your current sugar intake. Take note of foods and beverages high in added sugars that can be potential targets for reduction.

2. Educate Yourself:

- Understand the different names for added sugars (e.g., sucrose, high fructose corn syrup) and learn to identify them on nutrition labels. This knowledge will empower you to make informed choices.

3. Set Realistic Goals:

- Establish achievable, realistic goals for reducing sugar intake. Start

  with small, manageable changes to avoid feeling deprived or

  overwhelmed.

4. Identify High-Sugar Foods:

- Identify foods that are major sources of added sugars in your diet.

  This could include sugary snacks, sodas, desserts, and processed

  foods.

5. Gradual Reduction:

- Gradually reduce the amount of sugar in your diet by cutting back on

  one source at a time. For example, if you typically have two

  teaspoons of sugar in your coffee, try reducing it to one and

  eventually none.

6. Explore Natural Sweeteners:

- Experiment with natural sweeteners like honey, maple syrup, or stevia as alternatives to refined sugar. Be mindful of portion sizes and use them sparingly.

7. Choose Whole Foods:

- Opt for whole, unprocessed foods. Fruits, vegetables, lean proteins, and whole grains provide natural sweetness along with essential nutrients.

8. Read Labels:

- Get into the habit of reading nutrition labels when shopping. Look for products with little to no added sugars and choose those with simple, recognizable ingredients.

9. Meal Planning:

- Plan meals in advance, incorporating a variety of nutrient-dense, whole foods. This helps you make intentional choices and reduces reliance on processed, sugary options.

10. Stay Hydrated:

- Drink plenty of water throughout the day. Staying hydrated can help minimize cravings and support overall well-being.

11. Monitor Progress:

- Regularly assess your progress and celebrate small victories. Acknowledge the positive changes in your energy levels, mood, or taste preferences.

12. Seek Support:

- Share your no-sugar journey with friends, family, or a support group. Having a community to lean on can provide encouragement and motivation.

13. Be Patient and Flexible:

- Understand that changing habits takes time. Be patient with yourself and remain flexible, adjusting your approach as needed.

The gradual reduction approach recognizes that sustainable change occurs over time. By making mindful choices and progressively reducing sugar intake, individuals can create a lasting foundation for a healthier, no-sugar lifestyle.

Understanding the impact of sugar on health

Understanding the impact of sugar on health is crucial for making informed dietary choices. Here are key aspects of how sugar can affect the body:

1. Blood Sugar Levels:
   - Consuming foods high in refined sugars causes a rapid spike in blood sugar levels, leading to a subsequent crash. This can result in feelings of fatigue, irritability, and increased cravings.
2. Insulin Resistance:
   - Regularly high sugar intake may contribute to insulin resistance, a condition where the body's cells become less responsive to insulin. This is a precursor to type 2 diabetes.
3. Weight Gain:
   - Sugary foods and beverages are often high in calories but low in nutritional value. Excessive calorie intake from sugar can contribute to weight gain and obesity.
4. Inflammation:

- Chronic consumption of added sugars may lead to increased inflammation in the body, which is associated with various health issues, including heart disease and certain autoimmune conditions.

5. Liver Health:

   - Excess sugar, particularly fructose, is processed in the liver. Overconsumption can contribute to fatty liver disease, which may progress to more severe liver conditions.

6. Dental Health:

   - Sugar is a major contributor to tooth decay. Bacteria in the mouth feed on sugar, producing acids that erode tooth enamel and lead to cavities.

7. Heart Health:

   - A diet high in added sugars is linked to an increased risk of cardiovascular diseases. It can elevate blood pressure, triglycerides, and promote the development of atherosclerosis.

8. Mood and Mental Health:

   - Fluctuations in blood sugar levels can impact mood and energy levels. High sugar intake has been associated with an increased risk of depression and cognitive decline.

9. Addictive Properties:

   o Sugar can activate reward centers in the brain, leading to
     cravings and a potential addiction-like response. Breaking free
     from excessive sugar consumption may involve overcoming
     addictive tendencies.

10. Digestive Health:

   o Diets high in sugar can disrupt the balance of gut bacteria,
     potentially contributing to digestive issues. It may also increase
     the risk of developing conditions like irritable bowel syndrome
     (IBS).

Understanding these impacts underscores the importance of moderating sugar intake and choosing whole, nutrient-dense foods. Adopting a balanced diet that emphasizes fruits, vegetables, lean proteins, and whole grains can contribute to overall well-being and mitigate the negative effects associated with excessive sugar consumption. Regular consultation with healthcare professionals can provide personalized guidance based on individual health conditions and goals.

Health benefits of no sugar diet

Adopting a no-sugar diet can offer various health benefits, contributing to overall well-being. Here are some of the positive outcomes associated with reducing or eliminating added sugars from the diet:

1. Weight Management:
   - Lowering sugar intake can contribute to weight management by reducing calorie consumption and preventing excessive calorie storage as fat.
2. Improved Blood Sugar Control:
   - Eliminating or reducing added sugars helps stabilize blood sugar levels, reducing the risk of insulin resistance and type 2 diabetes.
3. Increased Energy Levels:
   - Without the energy fluctuations caused by sugar spikes and crashes, individuals on a no-sugar diet often experience more consistent energy levels throughout the day.
4. Enhanced Mood and Mental Clarity:

- Stable blood sugar levels can positively impact mood, concentration, and mental clarity, reducing the likelihood of mood swings and brain fog.

5. Reduced Inflammation:
    - Lower sugar intake is associated with decreased inflammation in the body, potentially lowering the risk of chronic diseases like heart disease and arthritis.

6. Improved Heart Health:
    - A no-sugar diet can contribute to better cardiovascular health by reducing the risk factors associated with heart disease, such as high blood pressure and elevated triglyceride levels.

7. Dental Health:
    - Eliminating added sugars helps maintain better oral health by reducing the risk of tooth decay and gum disease.

8. Enhanced Skin Health:
    - Lower sugar intake can contribute to clearer skin and may reduce the risk of skin conditions such as acne.

9. Better Digestive Health:
    - A no-sugar diet often includes more fiber-rich foods, promoting better digestion and a healthier gut microbiome.

10. Reduced Risk of Fatty Liver Disease:

   o Excessive sugar intake, particularly fructose, is linked to fatty liver disease. By eliminating added sugars, the risk of liver-related issues may decrease.

11. Lower Risk of Chronic Diseases:

   o Adopting a no-sugar diet may lower the risk of developing chronic diseases such as type 2 diabetes, certain cancers, and neurodegenerative conditions.

12. Increased Nutrient Intake:

   o Focusing on whole, nutrient-dense foods in a no-sugar diet ensures a higher intake of essential vitamins, minerals, and antioxidants.

13. Balanced Hormones:

   o Stable blood sugar levels contribute to balanced hormone production, positively impacting various bodily functions, including metabolism and stress response.

It's essential to note that individual responses may vary, and adopting a no-sugar diet should be approached with consideration for personal health conditions and dietary needs. Consulting with healthcare professionals or registered dietitians can provide personalized guidance and support on the journey to a healthier, lower-sugar lifestyle.

Meal plan

Certainly! Here's a sample one-day meal plan for someone on a no-sugar diet for beginners:

Breakfast:

- Scrambled Eggs with Vegetables:
    - Ingredients: Eggs, bell peppers, onions, spinach.
    - Preparation: Whisk eggs and cook with diced vegetables in olive oil.
- Whole Grain Avocado Toast:
    - Ingredients: Whole grain bread, avocado.

- Preparation: Toast the bread and spread mashed avocado on top.

- Fresh Berry Bowl:

  - Ingredients: Mixed berries (blueberries, strawberries).

  - Preparation: Rinse and mix fresh berries for a natural sweetness.

Mid-Morning Snack:

- Greek Yogurt with Nuts:

  - Ingredients: Plain Greek yogurt, almonds, walnuts.

  - Preparation: Mix a handful of nuts into the yogurt for added texture and flavor.

Lunch:

- Grilled Chicken Salad:

  - Ingredients: Grilled chicken breast, mixed greens, cherry tomatoes, cucumber.

  - Dressing: Olive oil, balsamic vinegar, lemon juice.

- Quinoa Salad:

  - Ingredients: Quinoa, diced bell peppers, black beans, cilantro.

  - Dressing: Lime juice, olive oil, salt, and pepper.

Afternoon Snack:

- Sliced Cucumber with Hummus:

  - Ingredients: Cucumber, hummus.

  - Preparation: Slice cucumber and dip in hummus.

Dinner:

- Baked Salmon with Roasted Vegetables:

  - Ingredients: Salmon fillet, broccoli, carrots, cauliflower.

  - Preparation: Season salmon and vegetables with herbs, olive oil, and bake.

- Cauliflower Rice:

  - Ingredients: Grated cauliflower, sautéed with garlic and olive oil.

- Steamed Asparagus:

  - Ingredients: Fresh asparagus spears, steamed until tender.

Evening Snack:

- Sliced Apple with Almond Butter:

    - Ingredients: Apple slices, natural almond butter.

Remember to drink plenty of water throughout the day to stay hydrated. This meal plan focuses on whole foods, lean proteins, and healthy fats, providing essential nutrients without added sugars. Adjust portion sizes based on individual caloric needs and consult with a healthcare professional or a registered dietitian for personalized advice.

No sugar diet drinks and beverages

When following a no-sugar diet, it's essential to choose beverages that are free or low in added sugars. Here are some no-sugar or low-sugar drink options:

1. Water:

- The healthiest and most hydrating option is plain water. Infuse it with slices of citrus fruits, berries, or cucumber for added flavor without added sugars.

2. Herbal Tea:

   - Herbal teas, such as peppermint, chamomile, or hibiscus, are naturally free of sugar. Enjoy them hot or cold without any sweeteners.

3. Black Coffee:

   - Black coffee without added sugar is a low-calorie and sugar-free option. If you enjoy a touch of sweetness, consider gradually reducing the amount until you can enjoy it unsweetened.

4. Green Tea:

   - Green tea is a healthy option that is naturally low in calories and sugar. It also provides antioxidants and other health benefits.

5. Sparkling Water:

   - Sparkling water, whether plain or flavored, can be a refreshing and sugar-free alternative to sodas. Check the labels to ensure no added sugars or artificial sweeteners are present.

6. Unsweetened Almond Milk or Coconut Milk:

- Unsweetened almond or coconut milk is a great non-dairy alternative. Ensure you choose the unsweetened varieties to avoid added sugars.

7. Vegetable Juice:

   - Freshly squeezed vegetable juices, like tomato or cucumber juice, can be nutrient-rich and low in sugar. Be cautious with fruit juices, as they can be high in natural sugars.

8. Iced Herbal Infusions:

   - Brew herbal teas, let them cool, and serve over ice for a refreshing, sugar-free beverage.

9. Kombucha (Check Labels):

   - Some kombucha brands offer low-sugar or no-sugar options. Check labels carefully, as some varieties can still contain added sugars.

10. Coconut Water:

    - Natural coconut water is a hydrating option with a subtle sweetness. Choose varieties without added sugars for a low-sugar beverage.

11. Homemade Smoothies:

- ○ Blend your own smoothies using unsweetened almond milk,
    fresh or frozen berries, greens, and a small amount of natural
    sweeteners like stevia or a ripe banana.
12. Lemon or Lime Water:
    - ○ Squeeze fresh lemon or lime into water for a citrusy flavor
      without added sugars.

Always read labels to ensure no hidden sugars or artificial sweeteners are present in seemingly "healthy" drinks. Gradually adapting to unsweetened options and appreciating the natural flavors of beverages can make the transition to a no-sugar diet more enjoyable

Frequently asked questions on no sugar diet for beginners

1. What is a no-sugar diet?

- A no-sugar diet involves avoiding added sugars and focusing on whole, unprocessed foods. It aims to reduce the consumption of refined sugars found in many processed and packaged products.

2. Can I eat fruits on a no-sugar diet?

- Yes, fruits are generally allowed on a no-sugar diet. They contain natural sugars along with essential nutrients and fiber. Moderation is key, and it's advisable to choose a variety of fruits.

3. Are natural sweeteners like honey allowed?

- Natural sweeteners like honey, maple syrup, or stevia can be included in moderation. However, the emphasis is on reducing overall sugar intake, including these alternatives.

4. How do I read food labels for hidden sugars?

- Check ingredient lists for terms like sucrose, high fructose corn syrup, and other sugar aliases. Pay attention to the total sugar content per serving and look for foods with minimal or no added sugars.

5. Is a no-sugar diet suitable for everyone?

- While many people benefit from reducing added sugars, individual needs vary. Pregnant or breastfeeding women, athletes, and those with specific health conditions should consult healthcare professionals for personalized advice.

6. What are some sugar-free snack options?

- Snack options can include fresh fruits, vegetables with hummus, nuts, seeds, and plain Greek yogurt. Choose whole, nutrient-dense foods to satisfy cravings without added sugars.

7. Can I still eat desserts on a no-sugar diet?

- Yes, you can enjoy desserts made with natural sweeteners like stevia, honey, or fruit. Experiment with recipes that use whole-food ingredients to create delicious, sugar-free treats.

8. Will I experience withdrawal symptoms?

- Some individuals may initially experience cravings or mood fluctuations when reducing sugar intake. Staying hydrated,

incorporating whole foods, and allowing time for adjustment can help
minimize these symptoms.

9. How can I handle social situations and dining out?

- Inform friends or hosts about your dietary preferences in advance.
  Choose wisely from restaurant menus, opt for grilled or roasted
  options, and ask for dressings or sauces on the side to control added
  sugars.

10. Can a no-sugar diet help with weight loss?

- Eliminating or reducing added sugars may contribute to weight loss
  by reducing overall calorie intake and stabilizing blood sugar levels.
  However, individual results vary, and a balanced approach to diet and
  exercise is crucial.

Always consult with healthcare professionals or a registered dietitian for
personalized advice based on individual health needs and goals.

Summary

Embarking on a no-sugar diet for beginners is a journey toward mindful and intentional eating, prioritizing whole, unprocessed foods. The essence of this lifestyle shift lies in understanding and minimizing the consumption of refined sugars, recognizing their pervasive presence in many processed foods.

In this dietary approach, individuals focus on nourishing their bodies with nutrient-dense whole foods, such as fresh fruits, vegetables, lean proteins, and whole grains. Natural sweeteners like honey or stevia may be incorporated in moderation as alternatives to refined sugar.

The journey begins with a gradual reduction in sugar intake, allowing for an adjustment period and making the transition more sustainable. Reading nutrition labels becomes a crucial skill, enabling individuals to identify hidden sugars and make informed choices while grocery shopping.

Balancing meals with a variety of whole foods ensures a rich supply of essential vitamins, minerals, and fiber. This approach promotes overall well-being, including improved digestion, sustained energy levels, and potential weight management.

The no-sugar diet is not about deprivation but about making empowered choices that align with health goals. It encourages mindfulness in eating, embracing the natural sweetness of whole foods, and finding creative ways to enjoy satisfying and delicious meals without relying on added sugars.

As beginners navigate this journey, they may discover increased energy, improved clarity of mind, and a sense of vitality. Support from friends, family, and community can further enhance the experience, creating a positive ripple effect that extends beyond individual choices.

Ultimately, the no-sugar diet for beginners is a pathway to a healthier lifestyle, fostering a deeper connection with food, and celebrating the abundance of nature's offerings. The journey is marked by a renewed appreciation for the simple yet profound sweetness found in the unadulterated goodness of whole, nourishing foods.

Conclusion

In the quiet serenity of that charming town, nestled amidst nature's embrace, Emma's journey towards a no-sugar diet blossomed into a transformative tale that resonated beyond her own kitchen. As the seasons changed, so did the rhythm of life in the community, echoing the subtle shifts in the choices made by those who had embraced Emma's wisdom.

Emma's story became a communal narrative—a shared experience of rediscovering the joys of whole, unprocessed foods. The town's marketplaces began to showcase an array of vibrant fruits and vegetables, local honey from nearby apiaries, and the fragrant aroma of whole-grain bread wafting through the air. The community gardens flourished, becoming a symbol of collective resilience and commitment to well-being.

One by one, neighbors embraced the no-sugar journey, not as a stringent set of rules but as a gentle awakening to the profound impact of mindful eating. Dinner conversations changed as families shared recipes, swapped tips on navigating the grocery store aisles, and celebrated the victories, big and small, in their quest for a healthier lifestyle.

Children, wide-eyed and curious, learned to appreciate the natural sweetness of a ripe peach or the crisp crunch of a carrot. Emma's kitchen became a hub of creativity, where cooking became an art, and the absence of refined sugar became an opportunity for culinary exploration. Baking sessions were infused with the fragrant notes of cinnamon and the earthy richness of whole-grain flours.

As the seasons cycled through their dance, the town's collective health and vitality began to tell a story of its own. Emma's initial steps toward a no-sugar diet had catalyzed a movement—a movement toward conscious choices and holistic well-being.

Friendship circles expanded beyond the bounds of backyards and picket fences as individuals, drawn by the allure of renewed energy and a clearer mind, joined hands in this communal quest for health. Community events transformed into celebrations of nourishing foods, where sugary temptations were replaced with bowls of fresh berries and platters of wholesome, homemade treats.

And so, the conclusion of Emma's story was not an endpoint but a continuation—a ripple in the fabric of community life that extended beyond her own journey. The echoes of her choices became a harmonious melody that resonated through every aisle of the grocery store, every dinner table, and every heart touched by the realization that embracing a no-sugar lifestyle was not a sacrifice but a gift—a gift of vitality, clarity, and shared well-being.

In that picturesque town, where the hills cradled stories untold, Emma's journey became a chapter etched into the collective memory—a reminder that every choice, no matter how small, can weave a tapestry of health, connecting hearts and homes in a melody of mindful living. And so, the town continued to thrive, its essence transformed by a simple yet profound decision: the decision to savor the sweetness of life without the need for refined sugar.